# My Food Allergy Journal

# If Lost, Return To:

_____

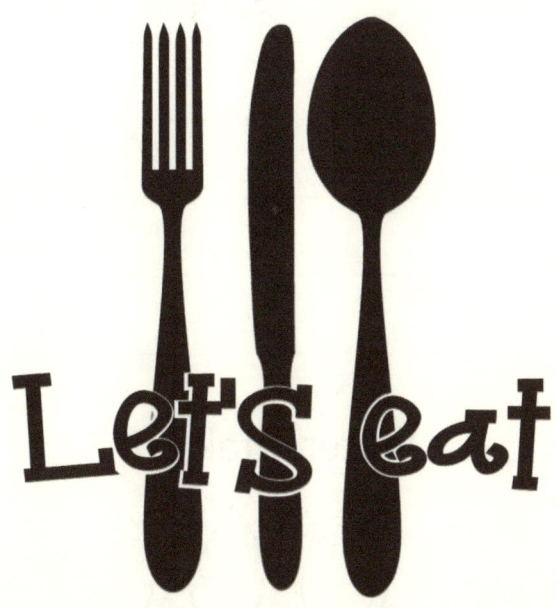

Date:_____

| Breakfast      Time: | Symptoms/Reactions |
|---|---|
| | |
| | |
| | |
| | |

| Lunch      Time: | Symptoms/Reactions |
|---|---|
| | |
| | |
| | |
| | |

| Dinner      Time: | Symptoms/Reactions |
|---|---|
| | |
| | |
| | |
| | |

## Water Intake:

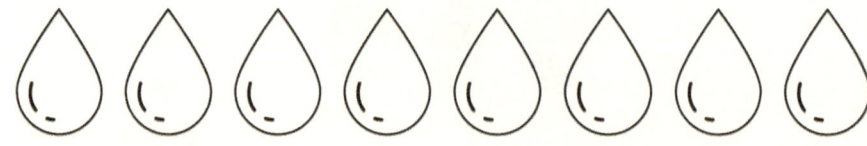

| Snack 1     Time: | Symptoms/Reactions |
|---|---|
| | |
| | |
| | |

| Snack 1     Time: | Symptoms/Reactions |
|---|---|
| | |
| | |
| | |

| Snack 1     Time: | Symptoms/Reactions |
|---|---|
| | |
| | |
| | |

## Notes:

_____

_____

_____

_____

_____

Date:_____

| Breakfast   Time: | Symptoms/Reactions |
|---|---|
|  |  |
|  |  |
|  |  |
|  |  |

| Lunch        Time: | Symptoms/Reactions |
|---|---|
|  |  |
|  |  |
|  |  |
|  |  |

| Dinner       Time: | Symptoms/Reactions |
|---|---|
|  |  |
|  |  |
|  |  |
|  |  |

## Water Intake:

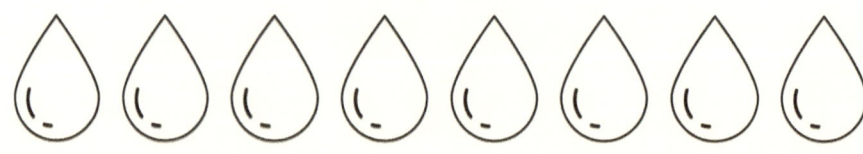

| Snack 1 Time: | Symptoms/Reactions |
|---|---|
| | |
| | |
| | |

| Snack 1 Time: | Symptoms/Reactions |
|---|---|
| | |
| | |
| | |

| Snack 1 Time: | Symptoms/Reactions |
|---|---|
| | |
| | |
| | |

## Notes:

_____

_____

_____

_____

_____

Date:_____

| Breakfast    Time: | Symptoms/Reactions |
|---|---|
| | |
| | |
| | |
| | |

| Lunch    Time: | Symptoms/Reactions |
|---|---|
| | |
| | |
| | |
| | |

| Dinner    Time: | Symptoms/Reactions |
|---|---|
| | |
| | |
| | |
| | |

## Water Intake:

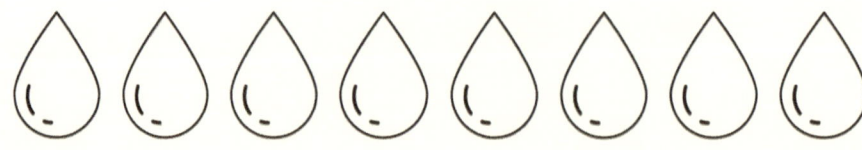

| Snack 1    Time: | Symptoms/Reactions |
|---|---|
| | |
| | |
| | |

| Snack 1    Time: | Symptoms/Reactions |
|---|---|
| | |
| | |
| | |

| Snack 1    Time: | Symptoms/Reactions |
|---|---|
| | |
| | |
| | |

## Notes:

_____

_____

_____

_____

_____

Date:_____

| Breakfast    Time: | Symptoms/Reactions |
|---|---|
|  |  |
|  |  |
|  |  |
|  |  |

| Lunch    Time: | Symptoms/Reactions |
|---|---|
|  |  |
|  |  |
|  |  |
|  |  |

| Dinner    Time: | Symptoms/Reactions |
|---|---|
|  |  |
|  |  |
|  |  |
|  |  |

## Water Intake:

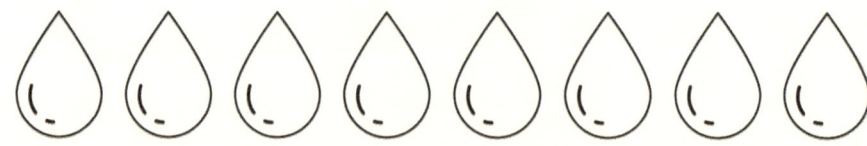

| Snack 1      Time: | Symptoms/Reactions |
|---|---|
| | |
| | |
| | |

| Snack 1      Time: | Symptoms/Reactions |
|---|---|
| | |
| | |
| | |

| Snack 1      Time: | Symptoms/Reactions |
|---|---|
| | |
| | |
| | |

## Notes:

_____

_____

_____

_____

_____

Date:_____

| Breakfast    Time: | Symptoms/Reactions |
|---|---|
| | |
| | |
| | |
| | |

| Lunch    Time: | Symptoms/Reactions |
|---|---|
| | |
| | |
| | |
| | |

| Dinner    Time: | Symptoms/Reactions |
|---|---|
| | |
| | |
| | |
| | |

## Water Intake:

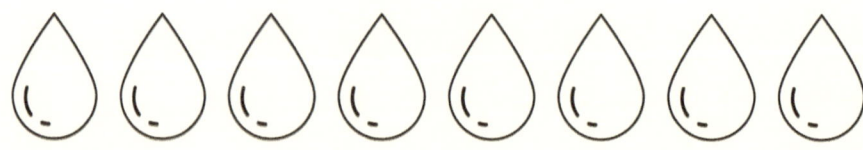

| Snack 1     Time: | Symptoms/Reactions |
|---|---|
| | |
| | |
| | |

| Snack 1     Time: | Symptoms/Reactions |
|---|---|
| | |
| | |
| | |

| Snack 1     Time: | Symptoms/Reactions |
|---|---|
| | |
| | |
| | |

## Notes:

_____

_____

_____

_____

_____

Date:_____

| Breakfast | Time: | Symptoms/Reactions |
|-----------|-------|--------------------|
|           |       |                    |
|           |       |                    |
|           |       |                    |
|           |       |                    |

| Lunch | Time: | Symptoms/Reactions |
|-------|-------|--------------------|
|       |       |                    |
|       |       |                    |
|       |       |                    |
|       |       |                    |

| Dinner | Time: | Symptoms/Reactions |
|--------|-------|--------------------|
|        |       |                    |
|        |       |                    |
|        |       |                    |
|        |       |                    |

## Water Intake:

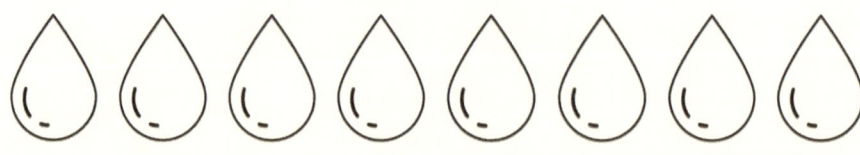

| Snack 1     Time: | Symptoms/Reactions |
|---|---|
|  |  |
|  |  |
|  |  |

| Snack 1     Time: | Symptoms/Reactions |
|---|---|
|  |  |
|  |  |
|  |  |

| Snack 1     Time: | Symptoms/Reactions |
|---|---|
|  |  |
|  |  |
|  |  |

## Notes:

_____

_____

_____

_____

_____

Date:_____

| Breakfast    Time: | Symptoms/Reactions |
|---|---|
|  |  |
|  |  |
|  |  |
|  |  |

| Lunch    Time: | Symptoms/Reactions |
|---|---|
|  |  |
|  |  |
|  |  |
|  |  |

| Dinner    Time: | Symptoms/Reactions |
|---|---|
|  |  |
|  |  |
|  |  |
|  |  |

## Water Intake:

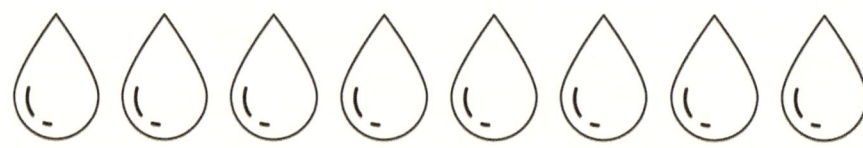

| Snack 1     Time: | Symptoms/Reactions |
|---|---|
|  |  |
|  |  |
|  |  |

| Snack 1     Time: | Symptoms/Reactions |
|---|---|
|  |  |
|  |  |
|  |  |

| Snack 1     Time: | Symptoms/Reactions |
|---|---|
|  |  |
|  |  |
|  |  |

## Notes:

_____

_____

_____

_____

_____

Date:_____

| Breakfast    Time: | Symptoms/Reactions |
|---|---|
| | |
| | |
| | |
| | |

| Lunch    Time: | Symptoms/Reactions |
|---|---|
| | |
| | |
| | |
| | |

| Dinner    Time: | Symptoms/Reactions |
|---|---|
| | |
| | |
| | |
| | |

## Water Intake:

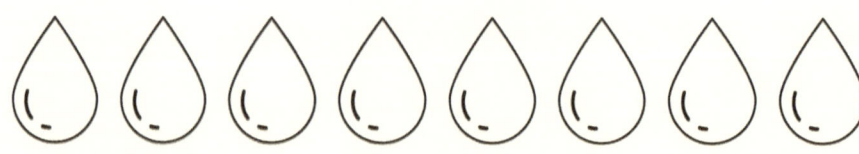

| Snack 1     Time: | Symptoms/Reactions |
|-------------------|--------------------|
|                   |                    |
|                   |                    |
|                   |                    |

| Snack 1     Time: | Symptoms/Reactions |
|-------------------|--------------------|
|                   |                    |
|                   |                    |
|                   |                    |

| Snack 1     Time: | Symptoms/Reactions |
|-------------------|--------------------|
|                   |                    |
|                   |                    |
|                   |                    |

## Notes:

_____

_____

_____

_____

_____

Date:_____

| Breakfast    Time: | Symptoms/Reactions |
|---|---|
| | |
| | |
| | |
| | |

| Lunch    Time: | Symptoms/Reactions |
|---|---|
| | |
| | |
| | |
| | |

| Dinner    Time: | Symptoms/Reactions |
|---|---|
| | |
| | |
| | |
| | |

## Water Intake:

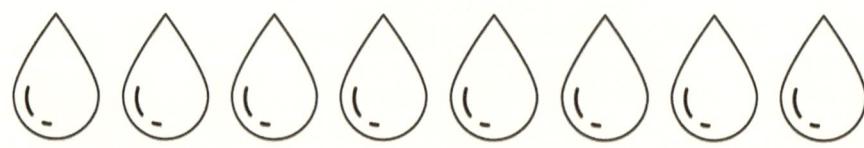

| Snack 1    Time: | Symptoms/Reactions |
|---|---|
| | |
| | |
| | |

| Snack 1    Time: | Symptoms/Reactions |
|---|---|
| | |
| | |
| | |

| Snack 1    Time: | Symptoms/Reactions |
|---|---|
| | |
| | |
| | |

## Notes:

_____

_____

_____

_____

_____

Date:_____

| Breakfast  Time: | Symptoms/Reactions |
|---|---|
|  |  |
|  |  |
|  |  |
|  |  |

| Lunch  Time: | Symptoms/Reactions |
|---|---|
|  |  |
|  |  |
|  |  |
|  |  |

| Dinner  Time: | Symptoms/Reactions |
|---|---|
|  |  |
|  |  |
|  |  |
|  |  |

## Water Intake:

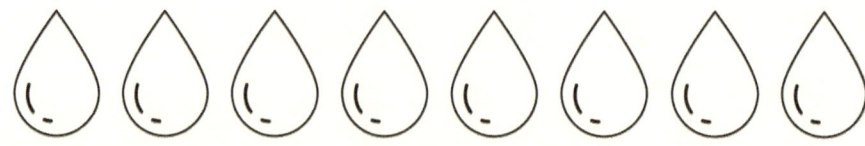

| Snack 1 Time: | Symptoms/Reactions |
|---|---|
|  |  |
|  |  |
|  |  |

| Snack 1 Time: | Symptoms/Reactions |
|---|---|
|  |  |
|  |  |
|  |  |

| Snack 1 Time: | Symptoms/Reactions |
|---|---|
|  |  |
|  |  |
|  |  |

## Notes:

_____

_____

_____

_____

_____

Date:_____

| Breakfast     Time: | Symptoms/Reactions |
|---|---|
| | |
| | |
| | |
| | |

| Lunch     Time: | Symptoms/Reactions |
|---|---|
| | |
| | |
| | |
| | |

| Dinner     Time: | Symptoms/Reactions |
|---|---|
| | |
| | |
| | |
| | |

## Water Intake:

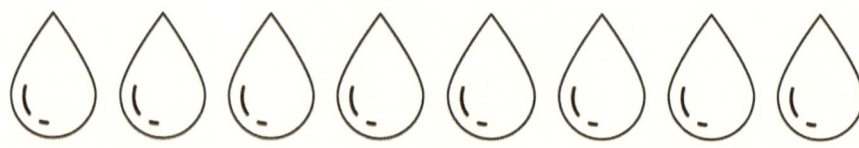

| Snack 1　　Time: | Symptoms/Reactions |
|---|---|
|  |  |
|  |  |
|  |  |

| Snack 1　　Time: | Symptoms/Reactions |
|---|---|
|  |  |
|  |  |
|  |  |

| Snack 1　　Time: | Symptoms/Reactions |
|---|---|
|  |  |
|  |  |
|  |  |

## Notes:

_____

_____

_____

_____

_____

Date:_____

| Breakfast        Time: | Symptoms/Reactions |
|---|---|
|  |  |
|  |  |
|  |  |
|  |  |

| Lunch        Time: | Symptoms/Reactions |
|---|---|
|  |  |
|  |  |
|  |  |
|  |  |

| Dinner        Time: | Symptoms/Reactions |
|---|---|
|  |  |
|  |  |
|  |  |
|  |  |

## Water Intake:

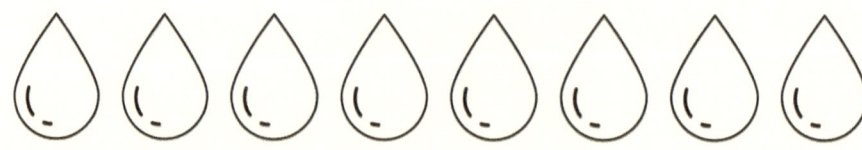

| Snack 1     Time: | Symptoms/Reactions |
|---|---|
|  |  |
|  |  |
|  |  |

| Snack 1     Time: | Symptoms/Reactions |
|---|---|
|  |  |
|  |  |
|  |  |

| Snack 1     Time: | Symptoms/Reactions |
|---|---|
|  |  |
|  |  |
|  |  |

## Notes:

_____

_____

_____

_____

_____

Date:_____

| Breakfast    Time: | Symptoms/Reactions |
|---|---|
|  |  |
|  |  |
|  |  |
|  |  |

| Lunch    Time: | Symptoms/Reactions |
|---|---|
|  |  |
|  |  |
|  |  |
|  |  |

| Dinner    Time: | Symptoms/Reactions |
|---|---|
|  |  |
|  |  |
|  |  |
|  |  |

## Water Intake:

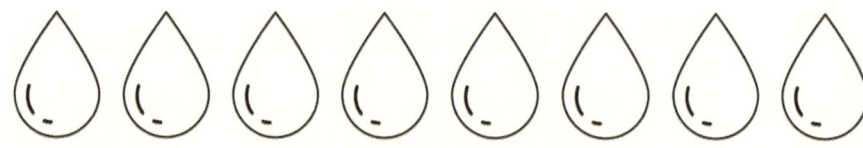

| Snack 1     Time: | Symptoms/Reactions |
|---|---|
| | |
| | |
| | |

| Snack 1     Time: | Symptoms/Reactions |
|---|---|
| | |
| | |
| | |

| Snack 1     Time: | Symptoms/Reactions |
|---|---|
| | |
| | |
| | |

## Notes:

_____

_____

_____

_____

_____

Date:_____

| Breakfast    Time: | Symptoms/Reactions |
|---|---|
| | |
| | |
| | |
| | |

| Lunch    Time: | Symptoms/Reactions |
|---|---|
| | |
| | |
| | |
| | |

| Dinner    Time: | Symptoms/Reactions |
|---|---|
| | |
| | |
| | |
| | |

## Water Intake:

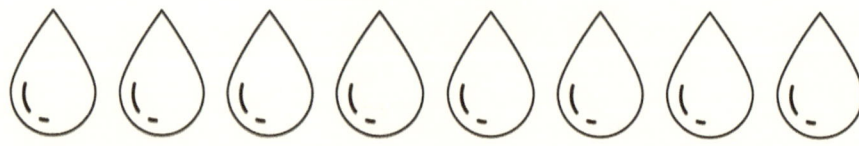

| Snack 1      Time: | Symptoms/Reactions |
|---|---|
|  |  |
|  |  |
|  |  |

| Snack 1      Time: | Symptoms/Reactions |
|---|---|
|  |  |
|  |  |
|  |  |

| Snack 1      Time: | Symptoms/Reactions |
|---|---|
|  |  |
|  |  |
|  |  |

## Notes:

_____

_____

_____

_____

_____

Date:_____

| Breakfast      Time: | Symptoms/Reactions |
|---|---|
|  |  |
|  |  |
|  |  |
|  |  |

| Lunch          Time: | Symptoms/Reactions |
|---|---|
|  |  |
|  |  |
|  |  |
|  |  |

| Dinner         Time: | Symptoms/Reactions |
|---|---|
|  |  |
|  |  |
|  |  |
|  |  |

## Water Intake:

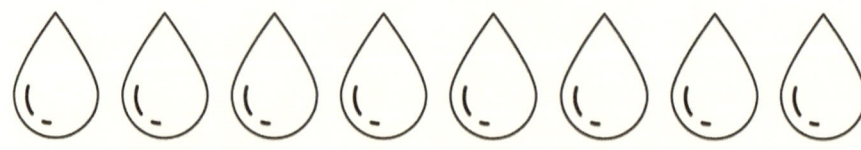

| Snack 1      Time: | Symptoms/Reactions |
|---|---|
| | |
| | |
| | |

| Snack 1      Time: | Symptoms/Reactions |
|---|---|
| | |
| | |
| | |

| Snack 1      Time: | Symptoms/Reactions |
|---|---|
| | |
| | |
| | |

## Notes:

_____

_____

_____

_____

_____

Date:_____

| Breakfast     Time: | Symptoms/Reactions |
|---|---|
|  |  |
|  |  |
|  |  |
|  |  |

| Lunch        Time: | Symptoms/Reactions |
|---|---|
|  |  |
|  |  |
|  |  |
|  |  |

| Dinner       Time: | Symptoms/Reactions |
|---|---|
|  |  |
|  |  |
|  |  |
|  |  |

## Water Intake:

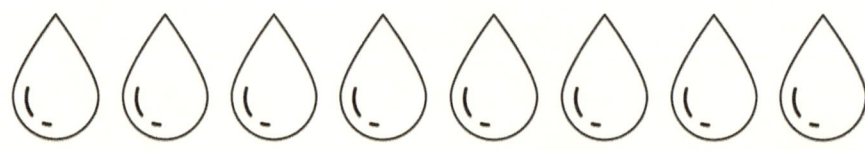

| Snack 1     Time: | Symptoms/Reactions |
|---|---|
|  |  |
|  |  |
|  |  |

| Snack 1     Time: | Symptoms/Reactions |
|---|---|
|  |  |
|  |  |
|  |  |

| Snack 1     Time: | Symptoms/Reactions |
|---|---|
|  |  |
|  |  |
|  |  |

## Notes:

_____

_____

_____

_____

_____

Date:_____

| Breakfast    Time: | Symptoms/Reactions |
|---|---|
|  |  |
|  |  |
|  |  |
|  |  |

| Lunch    Time: | Symptoms/Reactions |
|---|---|
|  |  |
|  |  |
|  |  |
|  |  |

| Dinner    Time: | Symptoms/Reactions |
|---|---|
|  |  |
|  |  |
|  |  |
|  |  |

## Water Intake:

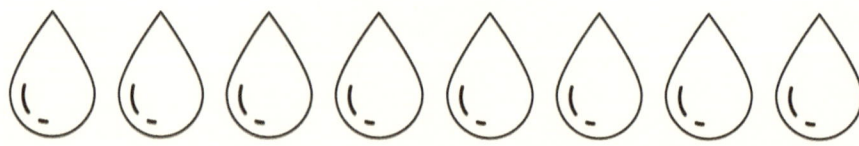

| Snack 1     Time: | Symptoms/Reactions |
|---|---|
|  |  |
|  |  |
|  |  |

| Snack 1     Time: | Symptoms/Reactions |
|---|---|
|  |  |
|  |  |
|  |  |

| Snack 1     Time: | Symptoms/Reactions |
|---|---|
|  |  |
|  |  |
|  |  |

## Notes:

_____

_____

_____

_____

_____

Date:_____

| Breakfast    Time: | Symptoms/Reactions |
|---|---|
|  |  |
|  |  |
|  |  |
|  |  |

| Lunch    Time: | Symptoms/Reactions |
|---|---|
|  |  |
|  |  |
|  |  |
|  |  |

| Dinner    Time: | Symptoms/Reactions |
|---|---|
|  |  |
|  |  |
|  |  |
|  |  |

## Water Intake:

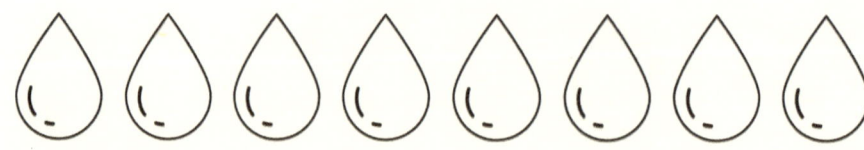

| Snack 1      Time: | Symptoms/Reactions |
|---|---|
| | |
| | |
| | |

| Snack 1      Time: | Symptoms/Reactions |
|---|---|
| | |
| | |
| | |

| Snack 1      Time: | Symptoms/Reactions |
|---|---|
| | |
| | |
| | |

## Notes:

_____

_____

_____

_____

_____

Date:_____

| Breakfast    Time: | Symptoms/Reactions |
|---|---|
|  |  |
|  |  |
|  |  |
|  |  |

| Lunch    Time: | Symptoms/Reactions |
|---|---|
|  |  |
|  |  |
|  |  |
|  |  |

| Dinner    Time: | Symptoms/Reactions |
|---|---|
|  |  |
|  |  |
|  |  |
|  |  |

## Water Intake:

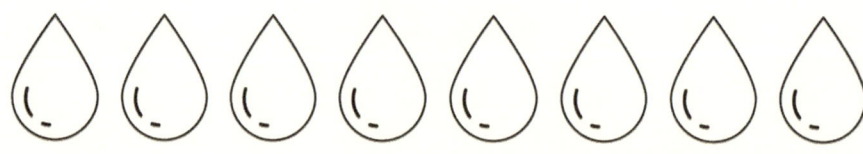

| Snack 1      Time: | Symptoms/Reactions |
|---|---|
|  |  |
|  |  |
|  |  |

| Snack 1      Time: | Symptoms/Reactions |
|---|---|
|  |  |
|  |  |
|  |  |

| Snack 1      Time: | Symptoms/Reactions |
|---|---|
|  |  |
|  |  |
|  |  |

# Notes:

_____

_____

_____

_____

_____

Date:_____

| Breakfast    Time: | Symptoms/Reactions |
|---|---|
|  |  |
|  |  |
|  |  |
|  |  |

| Lunch    Time: | Symptoms/Reactions |
|---|---|
|  |  |
|  |  |
|  |  |
|  |  |

| Dinner    Time: | Symptoms/Reactions |
|---|---|
|  |  |
|  |  |
|  |  |
|  |  |

## Water Intake:

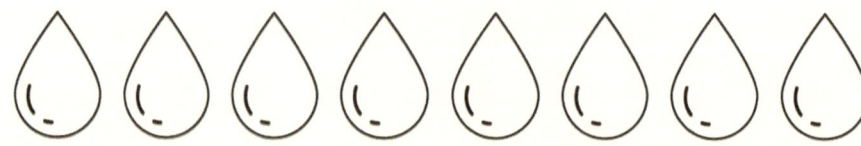

| Snack 1     Time: | Symptoms/Reactions |
| --- | --- |
|  |  |
|  |  |
|  |  |

| Snack 1     Time: | Symptoms/Reactions |
| --- | --- |
|  |  |
|  |  |
|  |  |

| Snack 1     Time: | Symptoms/Reactions |
| --- | --- |
|  |  |
|  |  |
|  |  |

## Notes:

_____

_____

_____

_____

_____

Date:_____

| Breakfast    Time: | Symptoms/Reactions |
|---|---|
|  |  |
|  |  |
|  |  |
|  |  |

| Lunch    Time: | Symptoms/Reactions |
|---|---|
|  |  |
|  |  |
|  |  |
|  |  |

| Dinner    Time: | Symptoms/Reactions |
|---|---|
|  |  |
|  |  |
|  |  |
|  |  |

## Water Intake:

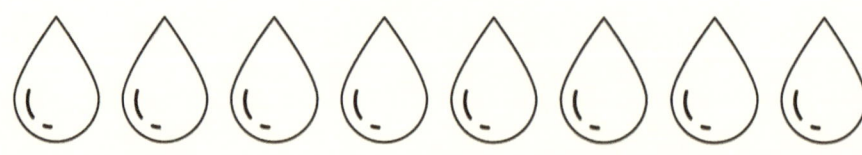

| Snack 1     Time: | Symptoms/Reactions |
|---|---|
| | |
| | |
| | |

| Snack 1     Time: | Symptoms/Reactions |
|---|---|
| | |
| | |
| | |

| Snack 1     Time: | Symptoms/Reactions |
|---|---|
| | |
| | |
| | |

## Notes:

_____

_____

_____

_____

_____

Date:_____

| Breakfast     Time: | Symptoms/Reactions |
|---|---|
|  |  |
|  |  |
|  |  |
|  |  |

| Lunch        Time: | Symptoms/Reactions |
|---|---|
|  |  |
|  |  |
|  |  |
|  |  |

| Dinner       Time: | Symptoms/Reactions |
|---|---|
|  |  |
|  |  |
|  |  |
|  |  |

## Water Intake:

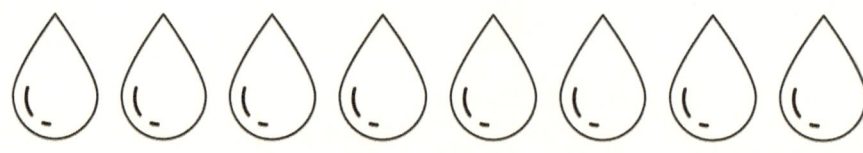

| Snack 1     Time: | Symptoms/Reactions |
|---|---|
| | |
| | |
| | |

| Snack 1     Time: | Symptoms/Reactions |
|---|---|
| | |
| | |
| | |

| Snack 1     Time: | Symptoms/Reactions |
|---|---|
| | |
| | |
| | |

## Notes:

_____

_____

_____

_____

_____

Date:_____

| Breakfast    Time: | Symptoms/Reactions |
|---|---|
| | |
| | |
| | |
| | |

| Lunch    Time: | Symptoms/Reactions |
|---|---|
| | |
| | |
| | |
| | |

| Dinner    Time: | Symptoms/Reactions |
|---|---|
| | |
| | |
| | |
| | |

## Water Intake:

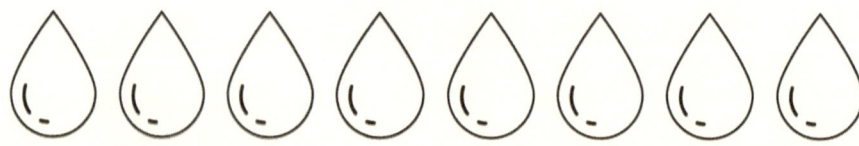

| Snack 1      Time: | Symptoms/Reactions |
|---|---|
|  |  |
|  |  |
|  |  |

| Snack 1      Time: | Symptoms/Reactions |
|---|---|
|  |  |
|  |  |
|  |  |

| Snack 1      Time: | Symptoms/Reactions |
|---|---|
|  |  |
|  |  |
|  |  |

## Notes:

_____

_____

_____

_____

_____

Date:_____

| Breakfast    Time: | Symptoms/Reactions |
|---|---|
| | |
| | |
| | |
| | |

| Lunch    Time: | Symptoms/Reactions |
|---|---|
| | |
| | |
| | |
| | |

| Dinner    Time: | Symptoms/Reactions |
|---|---|
| | |
| | |
| | |
| | |

## Water Intake:

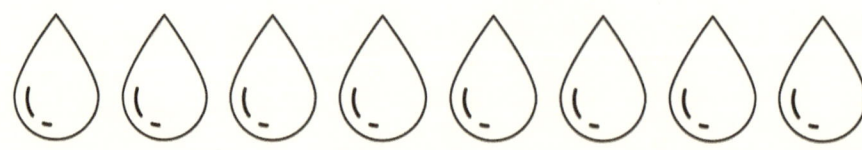

| Snack 1     Time: | Symptoms/Reactions |
|---|---|
| | |
| | |
| | |

| Snack 1     Time: | Symptoms/Reactions |
|---|---|
| | |
| | |
| | |

| Snack 1     Time: | Symptoms/Reactions |
|---|---|
| | |
| | |
| | |

## Notes:

Date:_____

| Breakfast    Time: | Symptoms/Reactions |
|---|---|
|  |  |
|  |  |
|  |  |
|  |  |

| Lunch    Time: | Symptoms/Reactions |
|---|---|
|  |  |
|  |  |
|  |  |
|  |  |

| Dinner    Time: | Symptoms/Reactions |
|---|---|
|  |  |
|  |  |
|  |  |
|  |  |

## Water Intake:

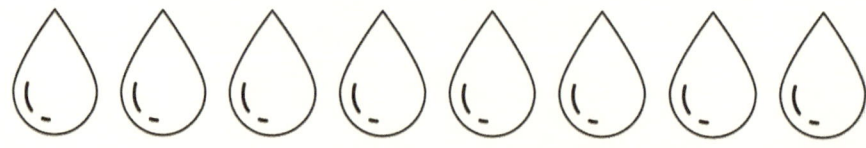

| Snack 1     Time: | Symptoms/Reactions |
|---|---|
|  |  |
|  |  |
|  |  |

| Snack 1     Time: | Symptoms/Reactions |
|---|---|
|  |  |
|  |  |
|  |  |

| Snack 1     Time: | Symptoms/Reactions |
|---|---|
|  |  |
|  |  |
|  |  |

## Notes:

_____

_____

_____

_____

_____

Date:_____

| Breakfast   Time: | Symptoms/Reactions |
|---|---|
|  |  |
|  |  |
|  |  |
|  |  |

| Lunch   Time: | Symptoms/Reactions |
|---|---|
|  |  |
|  |  |
|  |  |
|  |  |

| Dinner   Time: | Symptoms/Reactions |
|---|---|
|  |  |
|  |  |
|  |  |
|  |  |

## Water Intake:

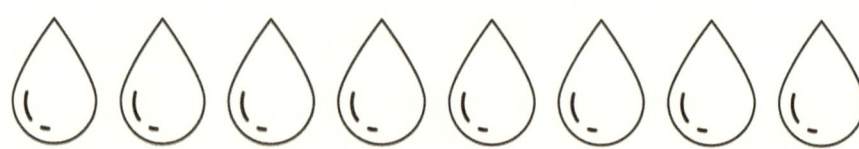

| Snack 1　　Time: | Symptoms/Reactions |
|---|---|
|  |  |
|  |  |
|  |  |

| Snack 1　　Time: | Symptoms/Reactions |
|---|---|
|  |  |
|  |  |
|  |  |

| Snack 1　　Time: | Symptoms/Reactions |
|---|---|
|  |  |
|  |  |
|  |  |

## Notes:

_____

_____

_____

_____

_____

Date:_____

| Breakfast     Time: | Symptoms/Reactions |
|---|---|
|  |  |
|  |  |
|  |  |
|  |  |

| Lunch     Time: | Symptoms/Reactions |
|---|---|
|  |  |
|  |  |
|  |  |
|  |  |

| Dinner     Time: | Symptoms/Reactions |
|---|---|
|  |  |
|  |  |
|  |  |
|  |  |

## Water Intake:

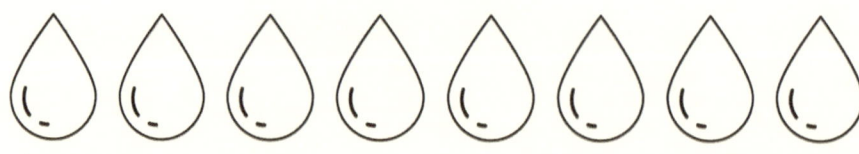

| Snack 1     Time: | Symptoms/Reactions |
|---|---|
|  |  |
|  |  |
|  |  |

| Snack 1     Time: | Symptoms/Reactions |
|---|---|
|  |  |
|  |  |
|  |  |

| Snack 1     Time: | Symptoms/Reactions |
|---|---|
|  |  |
|  |  |
|  |  |

## Notes:

_____

_____

_____

_____

_____

Date:_____

| Breakfast    Time: | Symptoms/Reactions |
|---|---|
| | |
| | |
| | |
| | |

| Lunch        Time: | Symptoms/Reactions |
|---|---|
| | |
| | |
| | |
| | |

| Dinner       Time: | Symptoms/Reactions |
|---|---|
| | |
| | |
| | |
| | |

## Water Intake:

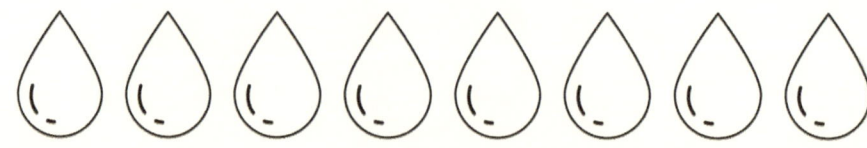

| Snack 1     Time: | Symptoms/Reactions |
|---|---|
| | |
| | |
| | |

| Snack 1     Time: | Symptoms/Reactions |
|---|---|
| | |
| | |
| | |

| Snack 1     Time: | Symptoms/Reactions |
|---|---|
| | |
| | |
| | |

## Notes:

_____

_____

_____

_____

_____

Date:_____

| Breakfast    Time: | Symptoms/Reactions |
|---|---|
|  |  |
|  |  |
|  |  |
|  |  |

| Lunch        Time: | Symptoms/Reactions |
|---|---|
|  |  |
|  |  |
|  |  |
|  |  |

| Dinner       Time: | Symptoms/Reactions |
|---|---|
|  |  |
|  |  |
|  |  |
|  |  |

## Water Intake:

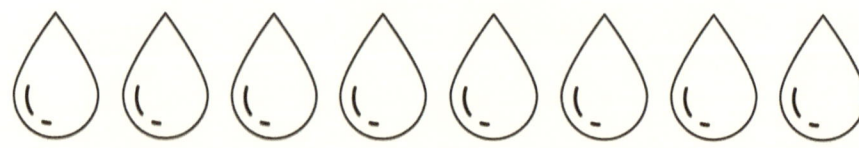

| Snack 1     Time: | Symptoms/Reactions |
|---|---|
|  |  |
|  |  |
|  |  |

| Snack 1     Time: | Symptoms/Reactions |
|---|---|
|  |  |
|  |  |
|  |  |

| Snack 1     Time: | Symptoms/Reactions |
|---|---|
|  |  |
|  |  |
|  |  |

## Notes:

_____

_____

_____

_____

_____

Date:_____

| Breakfast      Time: | Symptoms/Reactions |
|---|---|
|  |  |
|  |  |
|  |  |
|  |  |

| Lunch      Time: | Symptoms/Reactions |
|---|---|
|  |  |
|  |  |
|  |  |
|  |  |

| Dinner      Time: | Symptoms/Reactions |
|---|---|
|  |  |
|  |  |
|  |  |
|  |  |

## Water Intake:

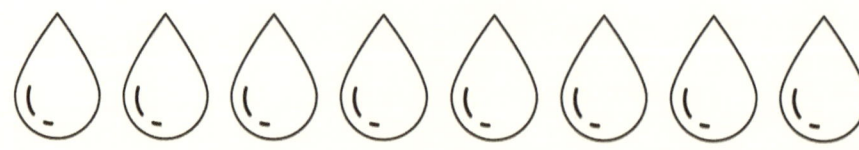

| Snack 1    Time: | Symptoms/Reactions |
|---|---|
|  |  |
|  |  |
|  |  |

| Snack 1    Time: | Symptoms/Reactions |
|---|---|
|  |  |
|  |  |
|  |  |

| Snack 1    Time: | Symptoms/Reactions |
|---|---|
|  |  |
|  |  |
|  |  |

## Notes:

_____

_____

_____

_____

_____

Date:_____

| Breakfast    Time: | Symptoms/Reactions |
|---|---|
|  |  |
|  |  |
|  |  |
|  |  |

| Lunch        Time: | Symptoms/Reactions |
|---|---|
|  |  |
|  |  |
|  |  |
|  |  |

| Dinner       Time: | Symptoms/Reactions |
|---|---|
|  |  |
|  |  |
|  |  |
|  |  |

## Water Intake:

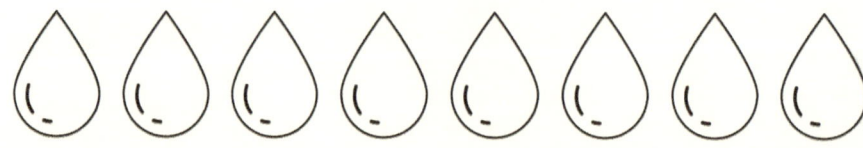

| Snack 1    Time: | Symptoms/Reactions |
|---|---|
| | |
| | |
| | |

| Snack 1    Time: | Symptoms/Reactions |
|---|---|
| | |
| | |
| | |

| Snack 1    Time: | Symptoms/Reactions |
|---|---|
| | |
| | |
| | |

## Notes:

_____

_____

_____

_____

_____

Date:_____

| Breakfast     Time: | Symptoms/Reactions |
| --- | --- |
|  |  |
|  |  |
|  |  |
|  |  |

| Lunch     Time: | Symptoms/Reactions |
| --- | --- |
|  |  |
|  |  |
|  |  |
|  |  |

| Dinner     Time: | Symptoms/Reactions |
| --- | --- |
|  |  |
|  |  |
|  |  |
|  |  |

## Water Intake:

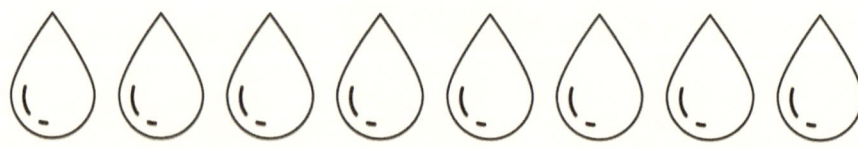

| Snack 1     Time: | Symptoms/Reactions |
|---|---|
| | |
| | |
| | |

| Snack 1     Time: | Symptoms/Reactions |
|---|---|
| | |
| | |
| | |

| Snack 1     Time: | Symptoms/Reactions |
|---|---|
| | |
| | |
| | |

## Notes:

_____

_____

_____

_____

_____

Date:_____

| Breakfast | Time: | Symptoms/Reactions |
|---|---|---|
|  |  |  |
|  |  |  |
|  |  |  |
|  |  |  |

| Lunch | Time: | Symptoms/Reactions |
|---|---|---|
|  |  |  |
|  |  |  |
|  |  |  |
|  |  |  |

| Dinner | Time: | Symptoms/Reactions |
|---|---|---|
|  |  |  |
|  |  |  |
|  |  |  |
|  |  |  |

## Water Intake:

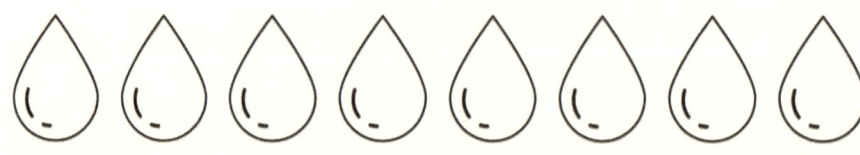

| Snack 1    Time: | Symptoms/Reactions |
|------------------|--------------------|
|                  |                    |
|                  |                    |
|                  |                    |

| Snack 1    Time: | Symptoms/Reactions |
|------------------|--------------------|
|                  |                    |
|                  |                    |
|                  |                    |

| Snack 1    Time: | Symptoms/Reactions |
|------------------|--------------------|
|                  |                    |
|                  |                    |
|                  |                    |

## Notes:

_____

_____

_____

_____

_____

_____

Date:_____

| Breakfast      Time: | Symptoms/Reactions |
|----------------------|--------------------|
|                      |                    |
|                      |                    |
|                      |                    |
|                      |                    |

| Lunch          Time: | Symptoms/Reactions |
|----------------------|--------------------|
|                      |                    |
|                      |                    |
|                      |                    |
|                      |                    |

| Dinner         Time: | Symptoms/Reactions |
|----------------------|--------------------|
|                      |                    |
|                      |                    |
|                      |                    |
|                      |                    |

## Water Intake:

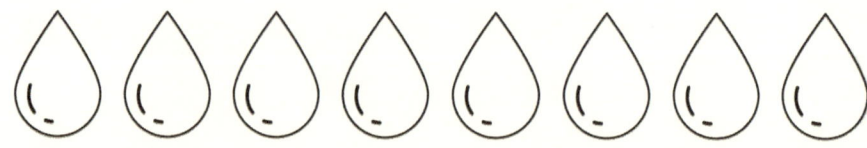

| Snack 1    Time: | Symptoms/Reactions |
|---|---|
|  |  |
|  |  |
|  |  |

| Snack 1    Time: | Symptoms/Reactions |
|---|---|
|  |  |
|  |  |
|  |  |

| Snack 1    Time: | Symptoms/Reactions |
|---|---|
|  |  |
|  |  |
|  |  |

## Notes:

_____

_____

_____

_____

_____

Date:_____

| Breakfast    Time: | Symptoms/Reactions |
|---|---|
|  |  |
|  |  |
|  |  |
|  |  |

| Lunch    Time: | Symptoms/Reactions |
|---|---|
|  |  |
|  |  |
|  |  |
|  |  |

| Dinner    Time: | Symptoms/Reactions |
|---|---|
|  |  |
|  |  |
|  |  |
|  |  |

## Water Intake:

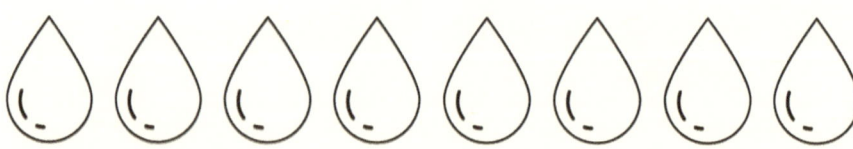

| Snack 1    Time: | Symptoms/Reactions |
|---|---|
|  |  |
|  |  |
|  |  |

| Snack 1    Time: | Symptoms/Reactions |
|---|---|
|  |  |
|  |  |
|  |  |

| Snack 1    Time: | Symptoms/Reactions |
|---|---|
|  |  |
|  |  |
|  |  |

## Notes:

Date:_____

| Breakfast    Time: | Symptoms/Reactions |
|---|---|
|  |  |
|  |  |
|  |  |
|  |  |

| Lunch    Time: | Symptoms/Reactions |
|---|---|
|  |  |
|  |  |
|  |  |
|  |  |

| Dinner    Time: | Symptoms/Reactions |
|---|---|
|  |  |
|  |  |
|  |  |
|  |  |

## Water Intake:

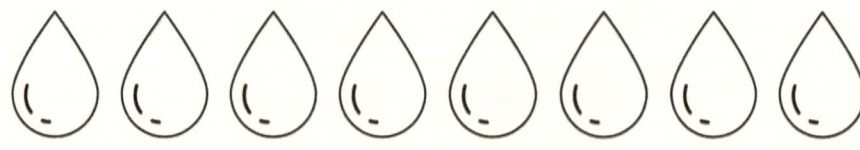

| Snack 1     Time: | Symptoms/Reactions |
|---|---|
|  |  |
|  |  |
|  |  |

| Snack 1     Time: | Symptoms/Reactions |
|---|---|
|  |  |
|  |  |
|  |  |

| Snack 1     Time: | Symptoms/Reactions |
|---|---|
|  |  |
|  |  |
|  |  |

## Notes:

_____

_____

_____

_____

_____

Date:_____

| Breakfast   Time: | Symptoms/Reactions |
|---|---|
|  |  |
|  |  |
|  |  |
|  |  |

| Lunch   Time: | Symptoms/Reactions |
|---|---|
|  |  |
|  |  |
|  |  |
|  |  |

| Dinner   Time: | Symptoms/Reactions |
|---|---|
|  |  |
|  |  |
|  |  |
|  |  |

## Water Intake:

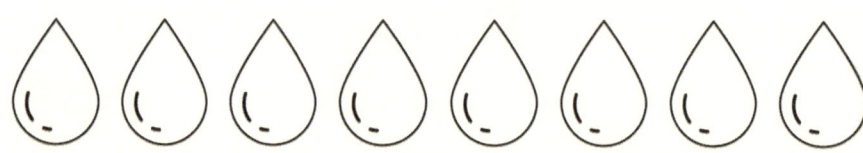

| Snack 1   Time: | Symptoms/Reactions |
|---|---|
|  |  |
|  |  |
|  |  |

| Snack 1   Time: | Symptoms/Reactions |
|---|---|
|  |  |
|  |  |
|  |  |

| Snack 1   Time: | Symptoms/Reactions |
|---|---|
|  |  |
|  |  |
|  |  |

## Notes:

_____

_____

_____

_____

_____

Date:_____

| Breakfast    Time: | Symptoms/Reactions |
|---|---|
|  |  |
|  |  |
|  |  |
|  |  |

| Lunch    Time: | Symptoms/Reactions |
|---|---|
|  |  |
|  |  |
|  |  |
|  |  |

| Dinner    Time: | Symptoms/Reactions |
|---|---|
|  |  |
|  |  |
|  |  |
|  |  |

## Water Intake:

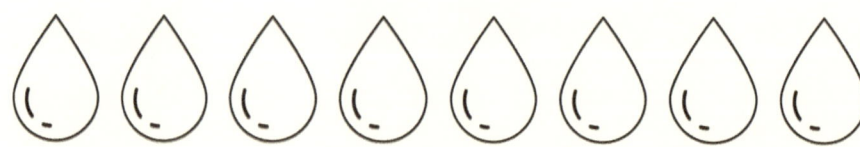

| Snack 1    Time: | Symptoms/Reactions |
|---|---|
|  |  |
|  |  |
|  |  |

| Snack 1    Time: | Symptoms/Reactions |
|---|---|
|  |  |
|  |  |
|  |  |

| Snack 1    Time: | Symptoms/Reactions |
|---|---|
|  |  |
|  |  |
|  |  |

## Notes:

_____

_____

_____

_____

_____

Date:_____

| Breakfast     Time: | Symptoms/Reactions |
|---|---|
|  |  |
|  |  |
|  |  |
|  |  |

| Lunch     Time: | Symptoms/Reactions |
|---|---|
|  |  |
|  |  |
|  |  |
|  |  |

| Dinner     Time: | Symptoms/Reactions |
|---|---|
|  |  |
|  |  |
|  |  |
|  |  |

## Water Intake:

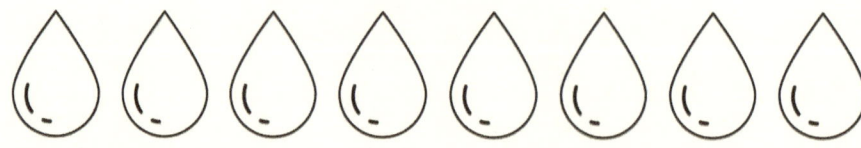

| Snack 1    Time: | Symptoms/Reactions |
|---|---|
|  |  |
|  |  |
|  |  |

| Snack 1    Time: | Symptoms/Reactions |
|---|---|
|  |  |
|  |  |
|  |  |

| Snack 1    Time: | Symptoms/Reactions |
|---|---|
|  |  |
|  |  |
|  |  |

## Notes:

_____

_____

_____

_____

_____

Date:_____

| Breakfast     Time: | Symptoms/Reactions |
|---|---|
|  |  |
|  |  |
|  |  |
|  |  |

| Lunch     Time: | Symptoms/Reactions |
|---|---|
|  |  |
|  |  |
|  |  |
|  |  |

| Dinner     Time: | Symptoms/Reactions |
|---|---|
|  |  |
|  |  |
|  |  |
|  |  |

## Water Intake:

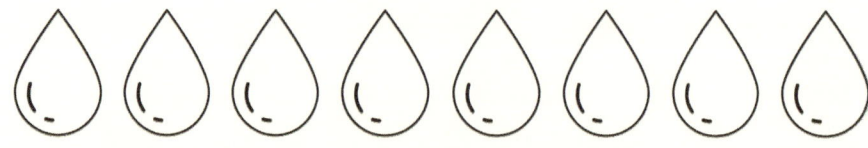

| Snack 1     Time: | Symptoms/Reactions |
| --- | --- |
|  |  |
|  |  |
|  |  |

| Snack 1     Time: | Symptoms/Reactions |
| --- | --- |
|  |  |
|  |  |
|  |  |

| Snack 1     Time: | Symptoms/Reactions |
| --- | --- |
|  |  |
|  |  |
|  |  |

## Notes:

_____

_____

_____

_____

_____

Date:_____

| Breakfast    Time: | Symptoms/Reactions |
|---|---|
|  |  |
|  |  |
|  |  |
|  |  |

| Lunch    Time: | Symptoms/Reactions |
|---|---|
|  |  |
|  |  |
|  |  |
|  |  |

| Dinner    Time: | Symptoms/Reactions |
|---|---|
|  |  |
|  |  |
|  |  |
|  |  |

## Water Intake:

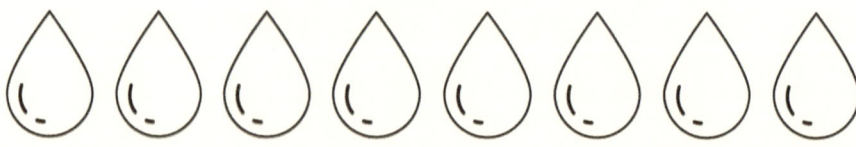

| Snack 1     Time: | Symptoms/Reactions |
|---|---|
| | |
| | |
| | |

| Snack 1     Time: | Symptoms/Reactions |
|---|---|
| | |
| | |
| | |

| Snack 1     Time: | Symptoms/Reactions |
|---|---|
| | |
| | |
| | |

## Notes:

_____

_____

_____

_____

_____

Date:_____

| Breakfast　Time: | Symptoms/Reactions |
|---|---|
| | |
| | |
| | |
| | |

| Lunch　Time: | Symptoms/Reactions |
|---|---|
| | |
| | |
| | |
| | |

| Dinner　Time: | Symptoms/Reactions |
|---|---|
| | |
| | |
| | |
| | |

## Water Intake:

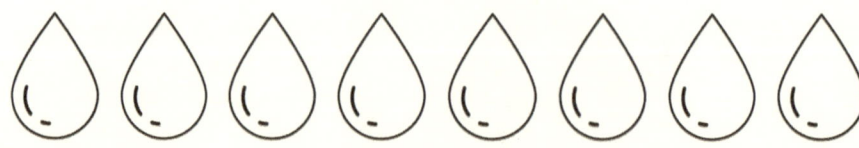

| Snack 1    Time: | Symptoms/Reactions |
|---|---|
| | |
| | |
| | |

| Snack 1    Time: | Symptoms/Reactions |
|---|---|
| | |
| | |
| | |

| Snack 1    Time: | Symptoms/Reactions |
|---|---|
| | |
| | |
| | |

## Notes:

_____

_____

_____

_____

_____

Date:_____

| Breakfast    Time: | Symptoms/Reactions |
|---|---|
|  |  |
|  |  |
|  |  |
|  |  |

| Lunch    Time: | Symptoms/Reactions |
|---|---|
|  |  |
|  |  |
|  |  |
|  |  |

| Dinner    Time: | Symptoms/Reactions |
|---|---|
|  |  |
|  |  |
|  |  |
|  |  |

## Water Intake:

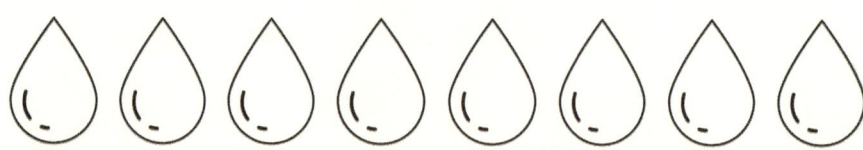

| Snack 1    Time: | Symptoms/Reactions |
|---|---|
|  |  |
|  |  |
|  |  |

| Snack 1    Time: | Symptoms/Reactions |
|---|---|
|  |  |
|  |  |
|  |  |

| Snack 1    Time: | Symptoms/Reactions |
|---|---|
|  |  |
|  |  |
|  |  |

## Notes:

_____

_____

_____

_____

_____

Date:_____

| Breakfast    Time: | Symptoms/Reactions |
|---|---|
|  |  |
|  |  |
|  |  |
|  |  |

| Lunch    Time: | Symptoms/Reactions |
|---|---|
|  |  |
|  |  |
|  |  |
|  |  |

| Dinner    Time: | Symptoms/Reactions |
|---|---|
|  |  |
|  |  |
|  |  |
|  |  |

## Water Intake:

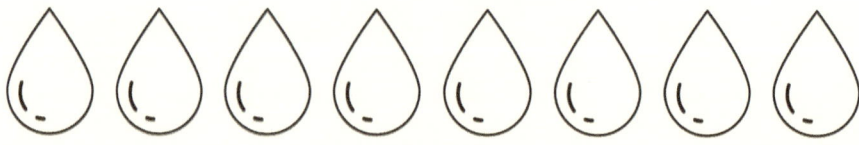

| Snack 1     Time: | Symptoms/Reactions |
|---|---|
| | |
| | |
| | |

| Snack 1     Time: | Symptoms/Reactions |
|---|---|
| | |
| | |
| | |

| Snack 1     Time: | Symptoms/Reactions |
|---|---|
| | |
| | |
| | |

## Notes:

_____

_____

_____

_____

_____

Date:_____

| Breakfast     Time: | Symptoms/Reactions |
|---------------------|--------------------|
|                     |                    |
|                     |                    |
|                     |                    |
|                     |                    |

| Lunch     Time: | Symptoms/Reactions |
|-----------------|--------------------|
|                 |                    |
|                 |                    |
|                 |                    |
|                 |                    |

| Dinner     Time: | Symptoms/Reactions |
|------------------|--------------------|
|                  |                    |
|                  |                    |
|                  |                    |
|                  |                    |

## Water Intake:

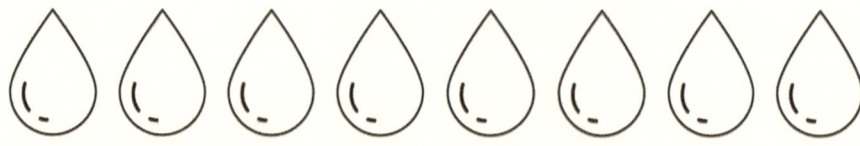

| Snack 1    Time: | Symptoms/Reactions |
|---|---|
|  |  |
|  |  |
|  |  |

| Snack 1    Time: | Symptoms/Reactions |
|---|---|
|  |  |
|  |  |
|  |  |

| Snack 1    Time: | Symptoms/Reactions |
|---|---|
|  |  |
|  |  |
|  |  |

## Notes:

_____

_____

_____

_____

_____

| GOOD FOOD | BAD FOOD |
| --- | --- |
| | |

| GOOD FOOD | BAD FOOD |
| --- | --- |
| | |

| GOOD FOOD | BAD FOOD |
| --- | --- |
|  |  |

| GOOD FOOD | BAD FOOD |
| --- | --- |
| | |

| GOOD FOOD | BAD FOOD |
| --- | --- |
| | |

| GOOD FOOD | BAD FOOD |
| --- | --- |
|  |  |